HEART DISEASE DIET RECIPES FOR SENIORS

"A healthy recipe book for heart disease patients"

TIM BROWN

TABLE OF CONTENT

CHAPTER 1

1. Describe Common Heart Disease Types

Heart illness encompasses a range of disorders affecting the anatomy and function of the heart. Heart valve disease, congenital heart abnormalities, arrhythmias, coronary artery disease, and heart failure are a few prevalent forms of heart illness.

- The most common kind, coronary artery disease, is characterized by reduced blood flow to the heart as a result of narrowing or blockage of the arteries supplying blood to the heart muscle, usually as a result of cholesterol and other material accumulation.

- Abnormal heartbeats, or arrhythmias, may result in diseases including bradycardia, tachycardia, or atrial fibrillation.

- Heart valve disease affects one or more heart valves, making it more difficult for the heart to pump blood efficiently.

- The inability of the heart to pump enough blood to fulfill the body's demands is referred to as heart failure.

- Congenital heart defects are structural issues with the heart that may damage the chambers, valves, or blood arteries present from birth.

2. Factors Affecting Seniors' Heart Disease

Age, family history, high blood pressure, high cholesterol, diabetes, obesity, physical inactivity, poor nutrition, excessive alcohol intake, smoking, and stress are some of the variables that might lead to the development of heart disease in seniors. The normal aging process may cause changes in the heart and blood arteries, which increases susceptibility to numerous heart-related disorders, including heart disease. As a result, seniors are more likely to acquire heart disease. Furthermore, a lifelong accumulation of risk factors may have a significant adverse effect on the cardiovascular system, raising the risk of heart disease.

3. Symptoms and Alert Signals to Be Aware of

Seniors with heart disease should be on the lookout for specific symptoms and warning signals. Chest pain or discomfort, palpitations, dizziness, lightheadedness, fainting, exhaustion, swelling in the legs, ankles, or feet, fast or irregular heartbeat, and trouble carrying out daily tasks are a few of these. Seniors need to be aware of these symptoms and should see a doctor right away if they exhibit any of these warning indicators.

4. Diet is Important for Managing Heart Disease

Because diet directly affects several heart disease risk factors, including high blood pressure, high cholesterol, and obesity, it is essential for controlling heart disease. Consuming fruits, vegetables, whole grains, lean proteins, and healthy fats is usually prioritized in a heart-healthy diet. In contrast, consuming processed foods, saturated and Tran's fats, salt, and added sweets is minimal. A diet like this may help manage weight, lower cholesterol, regulate blood pressure, and enhance heart health in general. A balanced diet may also promote general health and help with the better management of other illnesses like diabetes and obesity that are often linked to heart disease. To successfully treat heart disease in seniors, individualized dietary advice may be obtained via routine consultations with healthcare providers or trained dietitians.

CHAPTER 2

1. Nutrition's Function in Heart Health

Numerous nutrients are essential for lowering the risk of heart disease and supporting heart health. These consist of:

- Omega-3 fatty acids: Found in walnuts, flaxseeds, and fatty fish, these acids may lower triglyceride levels and reduce the risk of arrhythmias.
- Fiber: This nutrient, which can be found in whole grains, fruits, and vegetables, helps to maintain a healthy digestive tract and decrease cholesterol.
- Antioxidants: Found in fruits and vegetables, these compounds lessen oxidative stress and inflammation, which helps safeguard the heart.
- Potassium: This mineral, which may be found in foods like spinach, potatoes, and bananas, aids with blood pressure regulation.
- Magnesium: This mineral, present in leafy green vegetables, nuts, and seeds, promotes healthy muscular function and a regular heartbeat.

2. Crucial Elements of a Diet for Heart Health

The following vital elements should be the primary emphasis of a heart-healthy diet:

a. **Fruits and vegetables:** Packed with antioxidants, vitamins, and minerals, these foods promote heart health and lower the risk of heart disease.

b. **Whole grains:** They include fiber, vitamins, and minerals that assist in controlling cholesterol and blood pressure.

c. **Lean proteins:** Since they are low in saturated fat and may support heart health, lean protein sources include fish, poultry, lentils, and nuts.

d. **Healthy fats:** They may help decrease harmful cholesterol levels and the risk of heart disease. Examples of these include avocados, nuts, seeds, and olive oil.

3. Seniors' Portion Control and Balanced Meal Planning

For seniors to maintain a healthy weight and manage underlying medical disorders like diabetes and high blood pressure, portion management is essential. To prevent overindulging, seniors should try to eat smaller, more frequent meals throughout the day. A variety of nutrient-dense foods in sensible quantities, including a range of fruits, vegetables, whole grains, lean meats, and healthy fats, should be included in a balanced meal plan. Seniors should also know how many calories they consume and choose nutrient-dense meals that meet their daily calorie requirements while providing essential vitamins and minerals.

4. Advice on Adapting Well-Loved Recipes to Promote Heart Health

It is possible to adapt beloved dishes to promote heart health using several easy and efficient methods:

- Use herbs and spices to improve taste while reducing salt and sodium.

- Use healthier fat substitutes instead of saturated ones, such as olive oil in place of butter.

- Include more fruits and vegetables in your diet by adding them to salads, main meals, and side dishes.

- Select lean meat portions and trim off any excess fat before cooking.

- Replace processed grains with whole grains to boost your fiber intake and strengthen your heart.

- Swap out full-fat choices with plant-based or low-fat dairy products.

- Try to utilize as many fresh, healthy foods as you can instead of processed ones. Seniors may maintain a heart-healthy diet while still enjoying their favorite dishes by implementing these little changes.

CHAPTER 3

1. Advice for Filling Your Pantry with Heart-Healthy Items

Stocking a heart-healthy pantry should include a range of healthful and nutrient-dense essentials. Crucial pointers consist of:

- Opt for whole grains over refined grains, such as quinoa, brown rice, and whole wheat pasta.
- Add a range of dry beans, lentils, and legumes as great providers of fiber and plant-based protein.
- Choose canned foods with minimal salt content, such as beans, tomatoes, and fish, and rinse them before using them to reduce sodium.
- For good fats and protein, have an assortment of unsalted nuts, seeds, and nut butter on hand.
- To prepare and season salads, use heart-healthy oils such as avocado, canola, and olive oil.
- Keep a variety of herbs and spices on hand to enhance taste without using too much salt.

- Stock up on a range of frozen or canned fruits and vegetables to guarantee simple access to food even when fresh produce isn't accessible.

2. Important Kitchen Utensils and Equipment for Elderly-Friendly Cooking

Having equipment and accessories that make cooking easier and safer for seniors is crucial for enabling them to cook. Among the necessary kitchen equipment and tools are:

- Cookware and utensils that are lightweight and comfortable, reducing hand strain and improving grip for older adults with weak hands.
- Non-slip surfaces and cutting boards to avoid mishaps while chopping and prepping food.
- Easy-to-use and ergonomic kitchen gadgets that make meal preparation more accessible, such as food processors, blenders, and electric can openers.

- Comfortably raised workstations and worktops to suit wheelchair-using elders or those with mobility impairments.
- Simple storage options that are easy to reach and pull-out shelves, to reduce the amount of bending and reaching.

3. How Seniors Can Shop for Grocery & Make Healthier Decisions

Making heart-healthy food selections when grocery shopping is essential for seniors. Here are some pointers for wholesome food shopping:

- Making a list of items to buy before you go to the store can help you remain focused and prevent impulsive buys.
- Making whole grains, lean meats, and fresh vegetables a priority and avoiding processed and packaged meals heavy in sugar, salt, and harmful fats.
- Carefully reading food labels to ascertain the items' contents, nutritional value, and serving sizes.

- We are selecting items with minimum chemicals and preservatives, as well as low-sodium and low-sugar selections.

- Choosing lean meat and chicken portions, as well as omega-3-rich seafood like sardines, mackerel, and salmon.

- To guarantee a consistent supply of nutrient-dense foods, think about buying frozen or canned fruits and veggies that haven't had any added sugar or salt.

4. Knowing Labels and Making Knowledgeable Food Decisions

Making educated and healthful dietary decisions requires reading product labels. When reading food labels, keep the following in mind:

- Keeping an eye on serving sizes to guarantee that the nutritional value per serving is accurately understood.

- Examining the ingredient list to see whether artificial sweeteners, excessive sugar content, or bad fats are present.

- Keeping an eye on the serving sizes of sugar, salt, and saturated fat to prevent consuming too much of these potentially dangerous substances.

- Searching for goods that are rich in fiber and include healthy elements like antioxidants, vitamins, and minerals.

- Select goods with monounsaturated and polyunsaturated fats, butter substitutes, and little to no Tran's fats.

Recognizing and comprehending the particular standards that apply to claims made on labels, such as "low-fat," "reduced-sodium," or "sugar-free," to make well-informed choices. When making meal plans and grocery purchases, seniors may make more thoughtful and healthful decisions if they are aware of these labels.

CHAPTER 4

1. Healthy and Tasty Smoothies and Juices

Juices and smoothies may be a tasty and easy method for seniors to get the nutrients they need. When making delicious and nourishing smoothies and juices, keep the following in mind:

- To increase the consumption of vitamins, minerals, and antioxidants, include a range of fruits and vegetables, such as carrots, spinach, kale, and berries.
- To increase fullness and maintain the health of your muscles, include protein sources like Greek yogurt, almond butter, or chia seeds.
- Include heart-healthy components such as avocados, hemp seeds, or flaxseeds to boost the consumption of vital fatty acids and support cardiovascular health in general.

- To make the smoothie light and nutrient-dense, use low-fat milk, almond milk, or coconut water as the foundation.

- For a healthy choice, depend less on added sugars or sweeteners and more on the inherent sweetness of fruits.

2. Whole-grain and Low-Sodium Breakfast Options

A heart-healthy breakfast gives seniors the energy and nourishment they need to begin the day. Several whole-grain, low-sodium breakfast alternatives are as follows:

- Oatmeal or whole-grain cereals sprinkled with nuts, seeds, and fresh fruit to provide extra fiber, vitamins, and minerals.

- Avocado, eggs, low-sodium peanut butter, or low-sodium whole-grain bread or English muffins together for a filling and well-balanced dinner.

- A nutrient-dense breakfast choice is homemade muesli or granola prepared with whole grains, almonds, and dried fruits, served with low-fat yogurt or milk.

- A heart-healthy take on a traditional breakfast dish: whole-grain pancakes or waffles cooked with whole wheat flour and served with fresh fruit compote or sugar-free syrup.

3. Innovative and Tasty Yogurt and Oatmeal Recipes

Both yogurt and oatmeal are adaptable components that may be used in a wide range of tasty and inventive dishes. Here are some recipe suggestions for oats and yogurt:

a. For a quick and nutrient-dense breakfast alternative, try overnight oats prepared with rolled oats, yogurt, chia seeds, fresh fruits, nuts, and spices.

b. A filling and high-protein lunch may be made with a Greek yogurt parfait topped with granola, fresh berries, and a drizzle of honey or maple syrup.

c. Baked oatmeal cups with chopped nuts, cinnamon, and mashed bananas, which provide seniors with a quick and convenient breakfast choice.

d. Smoothie bowls made with yogurt and topped with fresh fruit, nuts, and seeds provide a visually pleasing, nutrient-dense breakfast choice with various tastes and textures.

Seniors may promote their overall heart health and well-being and have a pleasant and balanced start to the day by including these nutrient-dense, heart-healthy alternatives in their diet.

CHAPTER 5

1. Easy and Filling Salads Made with Heart-Healthy Foods

For seniors, salads may be a wholesome and cooling way to include heart-healthy foods in their diet. When making easy and filling salads, keep the following in mind:

- To provide vital vitamins, minerals, and fiber, start with a basis of leafy greens like spinach, kale, or mixed greens.

- Include a range of vibrant veggies, such as carrots, bell peppers, tomatoes, and cucumbers, to boost your intake of vital minerals and antioxidants.

- Include lean protein sources to enhance muscle health and encourage satiety, such as grilled chicken, salmon, or tofu.

- Add heart-healthy fats for taste and nutritional advantages from nuts, seeds, and avocado, among other sources.

- To improve the flavor without too much salt or sugar, use homemade vinaigrettes prepared with olive oil, balsamic vinegar, and fresh herbs.

2. Sandwiches and Wraps High in Protein and Low in Fat

For seniors searching for a heart-healthy dinner, sandwiches and wraps might be quick and filling. The following advice should be taken into account while making low-fat, high-protein sandwiches and wraps:

- Select whole-grain wraps or bread as your basis to boost your fiber intake and aid in improved digestion.
- To promote muscular function and deliver critical amino acids, include lean protein sources like turkey, chicken, and tuna or plant-based choices like hummus or grilled veggies.
- Add a range of fresh vegetables, such as sprouts, tomatoes, cucumbers, and lettuce, to provide taste and crunch, as well as essential vitamins and minerals.

- Choose healthier substitutes for high-fat condiments, such as homemade yogurt-based sauces, mustard, and low-fat or light mayonnaise.

- Go for lean cuts and low-fat cheese selections rather than processed meats and cheeses heavy in salt and saturated fat.

3. Healthy Stews and Soups Loaded with Vital Nutrients

Seniors may find comfort and nourishment in soups and stews, which provide a variety of vital elements. Take into account the following advice while making healthful soups and stews:

- To provide vitamins, minerals, and antioxidants, use a range of vegetables, including leafy greens, carrots, celery, and onions.

- To boost the protein content and encourage fullness, use lean protein sources such as skinless chicken, lentils, and beans.

- To lower the risk of high blood pressure and limit the salt level, use homemade or low-sodium broth.

- Include whole grains, such as quinoa, barley, or brown rice, to boost your fiber consumption and complex carbs.
- Use herbs and spices to season food to improve taste without using a lot of salt or extra sugar.

Seniors may enjoy a range of tasty and nourishing meals that promote their overall heart health and well-being by including these heart-healthy alternatives in their diet.

CHAPTER 6

1. Main Dishes Made Mostly of Vegetables and Low in Salt

Main meals made chiefly of vegetables may be tasty and heart-healthy, giving seniors a range of vital nutrients. Take into account the following advice while cooking delicious, low-sodium main meals that use vegetables:

a. Include a range of fresh or frozen veggies, such as spinach, broccoli, cauliflower, and bell peppers, to provide essential minerals, vitamins, and antioxidants.

b. Spices and herbs like paprika, garlic, ginger, and turmeric may improve the taste profile without using too much salt.

c. Incorporate plant-based protein sources, such as beans, lentils, and tofu, to increase fullness and provide a substantial amount of fiber and vital amino acids.

d. Try various cooking techniques, such as grilling, roasting, or sautéing, to enhance the veggies' inherent tastes and textures.

e. To boost fiber levels and make a more filling dish, add healthy grains like quinoa, brown rice, or whole wheat pasta.

2. Recipes Featuring Lean Protein and Mostly Fish and Poultry

A senior's diet may benefit from the tasty and heart-healthy inclusion of lean protein sources like fish and fowl. When cooking meals with lean protein, prioritize fish and poultry and take into account the following advice:

- Opt for fatty fish, such as trout, salmon, and mackerel, which are high in omega-3 fatty acids and may improve cardiovascular health by reducing the risk of heart disease.

- Choose skinless poultry, such as turkey breast or chicken, since they are lower in saturated fat and can be cooked in various ways, including baking, grilling, or poaching.

- Use a range of herbs, spices, and marinades to enhance taste instead of salt or fattening sauces.
- To make a well-rounded and nourishing dinner, serve with roasted sweet potatoes, steaming veggies, or a crisp salad on the side.

3. Easy and Delicious Whole-Grain Side Recipes

In addition to serving as a beautiful side dish to main meals, whole-grain foods are a rich source of fiber, vitamins, and minerals for seniors. The following advice should be kept in mind while producing straightforward and filling whole-grain side dishes:

- Pick a range of whole grains, such as faro, quinoa, brown rice, and barley, to improve digestion and enhance the consumption of complex carbs.
- To improve the taste profile without using too much butter or salt, add a mixture of dried or fresh herbs, lemon zest, or low-sodium vegetable broth.

- Add a range of veggies, such as bell peppers, carrots, or peas, to up the fiber content and make a nutrient-rich, eye-catching side dish.

- Try alternative cooking methods to add texture and variation to your meals, such as making cold grain salads, risotto, or pilaf.

- To make a gratifying and tasty whole-grain side dish, try adding nuts, seeds, or dried fruits.

Seniors may enjoy a wide variety of tasty meals that enhance their heart health and general well-being by including these heart-healthy alternatives in their diet.

CHAPTER 7

1. Ideas for Healthy and Low-Sugar Snacks for seniors

Healthy snacks help seniors maintain a healthy sugar consumption while giving them an energy boost between meals. Seniors should prioritize nutrient-dense snacks that provide prolonged energy and vital vitamins and minerals while thinking of healthy, low-sugar snack alternatives. Among the concepts are:

a. A small amount of unsalted nuts or seeds combined with fresh fruit slices or berries for a filling and healthy snack.

b. For a balanced and high-protein snack, try low-fat or Greek yogurt drizzled with honey, cinnamon, or oats.

c. Raw vegetable sticks, such as bell peppers, carrots, or cucumbers, served as a low-calorie, high-fiber snack with a side of hummus or Greek yogurt-based dip.

d. Homemade trail mix, which combines nuts, seeds, and dried fruits to create a portable, easy-to-eat snack that is nutrient-dense.

e. A light coating of nut butter or low-fat cheese over whole-grain crackers or rice cakes for a filling and well-balanced snack.

2. Recipes for Heart-Healthy Baking that Make Delicious Treats

While maintaining the wholesomeness and nutrition of the ingredients, baking may be a pleasurable and heart-healthy method to enjoy delights. Take into account the following advice while creating heart-healthy baking recipes:

a. Replace processed flours with whole-grain substitutes, such as almond, oat, or whole wheat flour, to boost fiber levels and provide vital nutrients.

b. To lower the total sugar level while increasing natural sweetness and taste, swap out refined sugars with natural sweeteners like honey, maple syrup, or mashed bananas.

c. Add heart-healthy fats to baked products, such as nut butter, avocados, or olive oil, to increase their nutritional content and promote heart health in general.

d. To lower the saturated fat and increase moisture in baked goods, use mashed fruits or unsweetened applesauce for oil or butter.

e. Try adding nuts, seeds, and dried fruits to baked items to give them more texture and crunch and to boost their nutritious richness.

3. Desserts & Sweets Made with Fruit and Less Sugar

Desserts made with fruit may provide a naturally sweet and nutrient-rich substitute for customary sugary sweets. When making fruit-based desserts and sugar-free candies, keep the following advice in mind:

- Add a range of frozen or fresh fruits, such as citrus fruits, apples, pears, and berries, to provide antioxidants, vitamins, and natural sweetness.

- Use a variety of vibrant fruits and add some citrus juice or cinnamon for taste and freshness when making fruit salads or fruit kebabs.

- To make an excellent and naturally sweet dessert alternative, make your fruit sorbets or frozen yogurt using ripe fruits and a little additional sugar.

- For a warm, cozy dessert that has less added sugar, bake fruit crisps or cobblers with oats, almonds, and a little bit of natural sweeteners.

- Make fruit-based jams, sauces, or compotes with minimum added sugar and natural thickeners to serve as a tasty and adaptable topping for a range of sweets and breakfast foods.

Seniors may promote their overall heart health and well-being while enjoying a range of delectable and gratifying snacks, sweets, and desserts by including these heart-healthy, low-sugar, and nutritional alternatives in their diet.

CHAPTER 8

1. Modifying Recipes to Meet the Dietary Needs of Seniors

Seniors with dietary restrictions must have their unique requirements and limits carefully considered when modifying recipes. When changing recipes for elderly individuals with nutritional requirements, keep the following in mind:

a. Find acceptable allergen replacements, such as gluten, dairy, or nuts, for those with dietary allergies or sensitivities.

b. For elderly individuals with diabetes, minimize the usage of refined carbs and added sugars and concentrate on regulating the amount of carbohydrates consumed by using low-glycemic index products.

c. To guarantee safe and easy swallowing for those with trouble swallowing or chewing, try adjusting the food's texture using purees, soft meals, or thickening agents.

d. Use substitute products and cooking techniques that satisfy the nutritional needs and cultural preferences of people with specific dietary or religious limitations.

2. Techniques for Regulating Consumption of Sugar and Sodium

Reducing sugar and salt consumption is essential for controlling heart disease and high blood pressure, among other medical disorders. Seniors may effectively reduce their consumption of sugar and salt by using the following strategies:

- Enhancing food flavors using fresh herbs, spices, and citrus juices rather than adding sugar or salt.
- Reducing the use of packaged and processed foods since they often have high added sugar and salt content.
- Carefully read food labels to find hidden sources of sugar and salt in items; wherever feasible, choose low-sodium or sugar-free alternatives.

- Promoting the eating of whole, unprocessed foods to lower intake of added sugars and hidden salt, such as fresh fruits, vegetables, lean meats, and whole grains.

- Preparing meals from scratch using entire, fresh ingredients to regulate better how much sugar and salt is added to the food.

3. Taking Care of Issues with Fats and Cholesterol

Seniors who want to lower their risk of heart disease and other cardiovascular issues must control their diet of fat and cholesterol. Seniors' worries about fats and cholesterol may be effectively addressed by using the following strategies:

a. Limiting the intake of red meat and processed meats rich in saturated fats and promoting the consumption of lean proteins such as chicken, fish, lentils, and tofu.

b. Including heart-healthy fats from nuts, seeds, avocados, and olive oil to support general heart health and encourage healthy cholesterol levels.

c. Promoting the intake of high-fiber foods to assist in improving digestive health and decrease cholesterol, such as fruits, vegetables, and whole grains.

d. Reducing the amount of Tran's fats and hydrogenated oils, which are included in processed and fried meals and may raise harmful cholesterol levels and cause heart disease, is advised.

e. Promoting consistent exercise and maintaining a healthy weight to control cholesterol levels and enhance cardiovascular health.

Seniors may improve their general health and well-being by putting these methods and modifications into practice, which will help them properly manage their dietary limitations, regulate their consumption of salt and sugar, and address their worries about fats and cholesterol.

CHAPTER 9

1. Seniors' Successful Meal Planning and Preparation Advice

A nutritious and well-balanced diet may be maintained by seniors with the support of adequate meal preparation and planning, which also guarantees accessibility and convenience to wholesome meals. Here are some pointers for seniors who want to prepare and arrange their meals successfully:

- Creating a weekly meal plan that consists of a range of foods high in nutrients, such as whole grains, fruits, vegetables, lean meats, and healthy fats.

- Making meals ahead of time and dividing them into manageable portions to guarantee that there is always access to a variety of well-balanced and healthful alternatives throughout the week.

- We employ practical kitchen gadgets, such as pressure cookers, slow cookers, and portion-sized cookware, to streamline meal preparation and improve organization.

- Using adaptable foods that may be prepared in several ways, encouraging creativity and experimentation in meal preparation.

- Labeling and labeling prepared foods and ingredients to guarantee freshness, stop food from going wrong, and make meal selection and consumption easier.

2. How to Include Exercise in Your Heart-Healthy Lifestyle

Engaging in regular physical exercise is crucial for preserving general health and heart health. The following are some tips for seniors looking to include training in a heart-healthy lifestyle:

- Speak with a medical expert or a trained fitness specialist to create a customized workout program that considers any physical restrictions and current health issues.

- Walking, swimming, or cycling are low-impact exercises that develop muscles and promote cardiovascular health without putting undue pressure on the joints.

- Engaging in strength training activities to increase muscular endurance and strength, which will enhance mobility and lower the risk of accidents and falls.

- Including stretches, yoga, tai chi, or other flexibility and balance exercises to improve joint flexibility, lessen stiffness, and increase stability and balance.

- Establishing reasonable and attainable fitness objectives and keeping a close eye on your progress can help you remain motivated and stick to your workout schedule.

3. Establishing Routines and Habits for Long-Term Heart-Healthy Eating

To maintain a healthy lifestyle and lower their risk of heart disease and its consequences, seniors must establish long-term heart-healthy dietary habits and routines. Seniors may adopt the following techniques to develop long-term, heart-healthy nutritional habits and practices:

- Creating a regular food plan with set mealtimes and nutrient-packed snacks to promote sustained blood sugar stability and high energy levels throughout the day.

- Creating a community and a shared responsibility for health and wellbeing by incorporating family members or caregivers in meal planning and preparation. This creates a helpful and encouraging atmosphere.

- Using mindful eating practices to improve digestion and reduce overindulgence, such as chewing food well, eating slowly, and enjoying the tastes and textures of each meal.

- Constantly educate oneself on the most recent dietary suggestions, nutritional standards, and healthy cooking methods to remain informed and make wise judgments about what to eat and how to prepare meals.

- To maintain diversity and avoid nutritional monotony, which may result in apathy and discontent with the meal plan, be flexible and open to introducing new foods, tastes, and dishes into the diet.

Seniors may develop long-lasting habits that support heart health and advance general physical and mental well-being by putting these techniques into practice and taking a holistic approach to health and wellbeing.

CONCLUSION

We have discussed various tactics, advice, and recipes designed to support senior heart health via the talks in this book. The groundwork for adopting successful dietary and lifestyle adjustments has been built by knowledge of the many forms of heart disease, the variables that contribute to its development, and the significance of a heart-healthy diet.

We have discussed the critical function nutrients play in maintaining heart health and the need to include these components in every meal. Additionally, we have included detailed instructions on how to choose kitchen utensils that are suited to your needs, fill your pantry with heart-healthy basics, and make wise decisions while grocery shopping. Seniors now have the information and skills to make heart-healthy eating choices by knowing how to read labels and modify their favorite meals.

Our investigation of a broad range of wholesome and delicious recipes—from juices and smoothies to main courses and desserts—has produced valuable and imaginative solutions that allow seniors to prioritize heart health while still enjoying tasty and filling meals. Furthermore, we have covered crucial tactics for handling dietary limitations, regulating the consumption of sugar and salt, and tackling issues about fats and cholesterol.

Finally, we have provided insightful advice on how to successfully prepare and plan meals, incorporate exercise into a heart-healthy lifestyle, and establish long-term, heart-healthy routines and eating habits. Seniors may start their road toward preserving ideal heart health, guaranteeing a higher quality of life, and promoting general well-being by considering these suggestions.